To Walk on Fertile Ground

KRISTI BROWN

TO WALK
ON FERTILE
GROUND

2008

To Walk on Fertile Ground

ACKNOWLEDGEMENTS

This book is so much more than a book. It is very much a glimpse through the windows of my soul. It is a place where many parts of me were formed early in my life and where many hurts and joys will indelibly remain in black and white so as to never be forgotten. It is a place where my soul has found acceptance with my imperfections and the freedom to embrace and share them with others who have searched for the meaning of their own lives.

It has been a lifelong dream to write this book, although I never imagined it to grow in the way it has—reflecting so many seasons of my life.

I know I must have many more lessons to learn along this journey I am blessed to call my own. I am who I am through lessons I've already learned but acknowledge with the deepest of emotions those who have walked near me on this pilgrimage. Some I have met along the way. Still others, I am learning, will join me as a sojourner.

Many people drifted into my life years ago like pollinated seeds that have been blown into a fertilized ground. Their purposes were all ordained, intentional, and planted in my life's garden. Still, there are many others who have helped cultivate my life along the path—teachers, colleagues, physicians, nurses, friends, and family. You have each helped to nurture, fertilize, till, mulch, and water my garden in some way so that I may bloom in the sun.

Thank you, Larry A., for teaching me so many things, but specifically how to craft my thoughts sequentially and the value of dreaming my dreams and putting them down on paper. Years ago you helped stoke the embers for writing this book that had all but burned out. I cannot imagine where this book would still be buried without your constant encouragement and prodding to write.

Gene Merkl—your daily prayers upon my life have humbled me beyond belief. "The Christ in me greets the Christ in you."

Dr. Jimmy Moore, thank you for not giving up on me. In so many ways, I owe my life to you, and there is not a day that goes by that I am not reminded of the healing path we walked together. You truly are living your calling, and I thank you for helping me to live mine.

My circle of friends, near and far—you know who you are, and I hope you will always know how much I cherish each of you for what you have brought to my life. Our moments of heartaches and triumphs, tears, and laughter so hard it hurts have lifted me to new heights. My life would not be my life without your touch on it.

Momma, words cannot begin to describe my undying gratitude to you—the woman who taught me to pull myself up. You have blessed me with an appreciation for writing, and the inspiration to write is your life's gift to me. You are the yardstick I use to measure the depths to which my soul will allow me to swim.

Lori, your lifelong desire to take care of those you love the most is an inspiration and a gift like no other. Our roots are part of the deep abundance we share as sisters. Forever.

Daddy, thank you for being you. Your independence has had more of a positive impact on my life than either of us could have imagined. I love you.

Teresa, there are no words to describe how grateful I am that our paths crossed. Because of your never-ending friendship, I know why we were both called to the same place once upon a time. Thanks for making me laugh every time we talk. Wheeeeeee!

Anne B., a fertile soul, who dared to hold onto me when the tides of this journey began swelling. I think of you every Mother's Day. I need a trip to SC.

To Sandra, what a mighty example of a mother you are. God's anointing is upon you, and I thank you for sharing your words of wisdom and your gift of ministry through the years. May you always know peace.

Pam E., you are one of the most unselfish individuals I have ever known. Your hands are a gift and your spirit moves my heart to places uncovered every time I am around you.

To my Chamber Institute colleagues—there are simply no words to convey my gratitude to you for sharing yourselves with me. Thank you for covering me in your thoughts and prayers. Thanks for the hats and visits, but, mostly, thank you for accepting me for who I am. I've learned so much from you all and wish you could see in my heart how I feel for each of you.

Marian, Ann, Rockin' Robyn, Kim, and Susan—thanks for being my sounding boards for everything crazy and wild to helping me conquer my doubts and insecurities. You are each strength personified in my mind and women of integrity. I have learned greatly from you.

To Robin, Dana, Tanner, and Grace—your friendship is something I always prayed for and it goes much deeper than being just neighbors. You have become a part of our family in so many ways from blowing our leaves, to sharing tomato pies, and sharing Christmas Eve and Christmas morning with us. I am a better person for knowing you and having you in my life, and I love you all so much.

Finally, to my entire family and my "in-loves"—for your love, prayers, understanding, acceptance, willingness to share yourselves with me and me with you, I thank you from the bottom of my heart. Suffice it to say, I would never have had the strength to complete this portion of my journey without your influence, love, and continual encouragement. I am forever changed because of you, and I pray that my life's garden will continue to offer an abundance of flowers to the world like those you have offered to me.

This book is dedicated to my beloved husband, Steve. You are my rock, my best friend, and the man with whom I am proud to be spending my life. (Thanks for asking!) You've lovingly given me that short course in country and have taught me how to stand up for myself with people who were weeds choking out the life in me. You've stood in the gap with me like no one in my life ever has and you've taught me what it means to live life passionately and to the fullest. You have loved me so deeply—flaws and all, and I cherish your faithfulness and your desire to take care of me. My rocking chair will always be next to yours—as will my heart. My mother gave me wings, but you've given me roots in this life we live together.

And just as the song played on the eve of our wedding, "...there's a family tree, surrounding me, reminding me that I do not stand alone...," I am reminded how much I love our own very special and deeply rooted family tree. And to all the women and families whose hearts ache and break silently through the ups and downs of infertility or cancer or any other hurt that is too deep to speak of, may

*you always know you are never alone in your journey.
Every cut of the spade, every turn of the dirt, every drought
and flood are nourishments for your garden in life.
I dedicate the pages of this book to you, the reader, and
I pray you will find a light heart, peace, joy, and a
knowledge that you too "walk on fertile ground."*

For "Katie"

INTRODUCTION

For two hours, I have been lying awake—toss, turn, toss. Sigh. Toss and turn some more. Twice I've replayed and listened to my CD, specially designed with music that should induce sleep. It usually helps. But tonight? Of course—not tonight. I'm finally convinced that the quiet stirring and restlessness in my head and my heart is the Lord. "Get up, silly! I've got words for you."

My home is eerily silent on this cold December night. My husband is hunting in Illinois for the weekend and will return tomorrow. My two Labrador retrievers are snoring quietly after a long day of play, and the Christmas tree lights beckon me just to sit in awe of their quiet warmth. I cannot linger long in thought, though, because my head is keeping a much swifter pace than I dare to imagine. It's been far too long that I've had words to write. Words that actually mean something and carry with them the essence of heart and soul sometimes don't come as easily for a writer as one would imagine.

Do I even dare to call myself an author? In so many ways, I'm simply following my heart to complete this project. But in truth, I have always thought of myself as an author. My seventh-grade English teacher planted the seed in me so long ago to develop my words creatively. Conversely, the following year my eighth-grade English teacher took me to a Wordsmith competition where I froze up and could not allow myself to think or develop creatively—and I stopped writing. A college creative writing professor loved one of my stories enough that his encouraging words began to force back to the surface my vision for writing.

Much like the fact that it sometimes takes bamboo many years to establish itself and grow, in my dreams, I have dared to imagine that one day I would write a book.

Though I've never been able to describe or to visualize totally the exact type of book, I've always known somehow, someday, it would come to fruition.

That day is now, and I pray for all who are led to this book—perhaps from a friend, a family member, or even by accident, that you will find peace and encouragement as I have found through my journey.

Each step along the way, I've learned, has been purposeful for the lessons gained on this path. Each footprint left behind has been but an outline of where I have been and where I am going. It has taken me a long time to realize, understand, believe, and to experience fully that I have never been all alone in my life's journey. God, through His mercy and divine grace, chose *me* as His child many years ago and it is He who has truly carried me all this way. As I begin tonight, this book is no exception to the journey.

If this book were a painting of my life, you would see that each detail is a colored stroke of genius painted by the Almighty Artist, our Heavenly Father. My intent is to encourage you to know, without a doubt, that it is God's infinite mercy and grace that is showered upon each of us every single day. Regardless of where we are in our lives, what hurts we are burdened by, what accomplishments are tagged by our names, or what type of ground we've claimed for ourselves, hope prevails in us all.

Whether you are just starting out, eager and ready to change the world, or are struggling with the complexities of life, this book is for you. If you are considering a career change, perhaps embarking on a new relationship, or raising a family in a two-income home, my message to you is simple: consider where you are *right now* as your garden—a place to where you are being led. Do not wish your life away as it is now, hoping for healing, a way out, a way in, or for the next big opportunity. I want you to know that whatever struggles or joys you face are an important part of where you will be a month, a year, and ten years from now. Each step on the path and every ounce of rain and sun are vital to understanding your purpose in this life.

Don't we all question that at some point? Shouldn't we all grasp onto that inner voice that tells us we are to become more than who we are and that life is about more than ourselves?

Once we get that lesson, embrace it, and understand that life is "not about me," only then will we live in abundant joy and begin to walk on fertile ground.

Now it is God who makes both us and you stand firm in Christ.
He anointed us, set His seal of ownership on us,
and put His Spirit in our hearts as a deposit,
guaranteeing what is to come.

2 Corinthians 1:21-22

CHAPTER 1

As I pull into the tree-covered drive of our home, I look in exasperation at what lies before me. The drive up is actually quite nice, a little curve to the right and a slight bend to the left up to the broken concrete parking pad. I sit in my Toyota 4Runner facing the corner of the house and once again roll my eyes to see the cracks in the brick façade and between the mortar and wonder how in the world our house is even still standing.

It's no surprise because we live in one of the worst parts of the county for foundation problems. The soil in our part of the state is a clay consistency that reminds me of what I used to play with in pre-kindergarten Sunday school except mixed with a smell of pure stench.

There are no aeration opportunities at all below the top layer, so the clay bulk clumps as the ground expands when it's wet and compresses tightly when the drought-like days of summer force cracks so wide in our lawn you almost have to jump over them. Over time, whatever stands on this type of ground cracks too unless the foundation is prepared properly.

Pushing it out of my mind, I walk inside and am greeted eagerly by our two yellow Labrador retrievers, Sadie and Lily, and quickly forget about all the repairs we need to make to our home that is obviously shifting with the clay below it.

The immediate need at this moment is for them to go outside. After a ten-hour workday away, I feel terrible; they've been home that long without us to play with them or take them out. But they don't seem to mind. All they desire is to run and bounce, stop to use the bathroom, grab a Frisbee or ball, and play, play, play. Unconditional love—there's nothing that compares.

So we follow our usual end-of-the-day routine of playing, potty break, and suppertime before escaping into the fabulously cool house far away from the annoying mosquitoes and pesky horseflies that share our five acres.

My dogs live in the present, the here and now. An hour ago no longer matters and an hour from now doesn't belong to them yet. That's the lesson of the day. That's the gift I was recently given, and one I want to share with you.

Journey with me up this driveway, if you will. Look into the window to my soul, and then imagine an abundant harvest for your own life.

"For I know the plans I have for you," declares the Lord,
"plans to prosper you and not to harm you,
plans to give you hope and a future."

Jeremiah 29:11

CHAPTER 2

It is truly a miracle that I am where I am today. God's grace has always been prevalent in my heart. Sometimes I am not sure I understand why I was chosen to be as blessed as I have been in my life, or as blessed as I am now. God, or at least the knowledge of Him, has always been present in my life—even if He was as faintly heard as a deer that tenderly slips to drink from a stream.

As a young Christian, I never really allowed myself to understand all the things that knowing God could mean for my life. Growing up, I could not fathom or begin to understand all the blessings He had stored up for me or why He had them ready for me at all.

All the blessings I surely missed out on because of pure ignorance or selfishness, somehow turned into years of not only spiritual distance from failures and missteps, but also fun times, laughter, and honest attempts at trying to be the best person I could possibly be. I once thought it was all about me. I find it amazing and inspiring that children so many years younger than I have experienced a truer sense of Christ so much earlier in their lives than I ever dared to believe could be possible for me as a child. Their commitment to living a Christ-centered life surely must have been brought to them through the grace that much in the same way has entered my life in adulthood. I pray for their innocence, that life will not be so harsh to their gardens, and that the grounds they walk will remain steadfast and proliferate.

In retrospect, I also know now that God's plan for me has been purposeful and it has been a part of His plan for me to learn these life lessons just as I have had to learn them. A gardener knows that a fruitful and bountiful garden must be prepared deeply below the surface. Tilling, fertilizing, and a lot of watering yields bouquets or baskets full of the harvest.

I suppose I could begin this journey with you early on in my life. I was saved when I was nine, and I cannot really remember a time not knowing the Lord or knowing that His plan is to be our purpose in life. However, I was never discipled growing up, and eventually I just went through the motions of adolescence, complacent in the knowledge that I was saved, but not truly knowing God.

My parents divorced when I was very young. My mother remarried and divorced twice more. Though I sometimes longed for a "normal" life, I learned from her how deeply families are affected by broken relationships and lost loves, and how our choices in life are always met with positive and negative reactions on those around us. Those broken relationships instilled in me a hope that I could have a different life. I set my mind in those early years to dedicate myself to my commitments and to do my part to make sure I contributed to a healthy marriage and family.

I also learned from her how much a mother loves, or should love, her children. She taught me the meaning of sacrifice, the beauty of true joy, and perseverance. She is, in my humble opinion, a "steel magnolia"—as aptly described and played out in that wonderful movie. For my sister and me, she would give us her all to let us know we were loved.

Though I didn't know how to verbalize it, I felt awkward in my skin. Growing up, I spent many years wondering if anyone else felt the same way I did. For years, I suppressed my disappointment with life and relationships and neglected dealing with it. Perhaps I did not know how to "weed my garden"—no one had ever given me a spade or shears or even permission to get down on my knees and dig out the unwanted blades of grass. And I've come to realize how our minds work is a reflection of our familial environments and our family roots.

I remember being determined from a very early age to be different from anyone else in my family; I *would* survive the storms of life and do it better than most. I was twelve when I came face to face with Satan as I stood over a loved one's hospital bed while she recovered from an attempted suicide. I realized what a thief he is—wanting to rob us of our happiness, our lives, ourselves.

I did not know then how much that moment would change me. I was deeply influenced by and acutely aware of the fact that whatever I did from that point on, others would be impacted either positively or negatively. And I strove to "do good".

I determined in my mind and in my heart that I would not repeat family behaviors and allow crises to let me get so low that there was no other way out. I later realized I had made up my mind to be what is oftentimes referred to as a transitional person—someone who breaks those ties that bind. But most importantly, I learned the value of life—what it means to be loved, to love, to hurt, to need someone to understand me, to feel that I belong and am accepted.

But I also have realized that Satan finds a way very early in our lives to convince us that we alone are capable of controlling our lives all by ourselves. He does not discriminate in planting this concept, and we are all susceptible to his deceitfulness. Looking back, I've always had a deep-seated need for approval and wanted earnestly to please those around me. Getting good grades, working at part-time jobs when friends were on spring break, going to and graduating from college with honors were a part of my internal beacon. If I could *achieve* things, as the world told me and every other teenager we should, then I would be successful. Approved. Whole.

Satan takes the opportunities that are meant to build our character and twists the circumstances in our minds so that we actually begin to believe *we* alone are in complete control of everything in our lives—good and bad. That happened to me. I felt alone in the world—and that I had to depend on only myself for my happiness, my success, my life.

But somewhere along the way, and by His grace, God continued to whisper promises to me. "You are mine and I am going to show you how much I love you." Don't misunderstand. Our lives mirror what we give to them and hard work does pay off. But the questions no longer exist when we embrace and live through faith.

And so the plowing of the grounds begins.

Have you not put a hedge around him and his household and everything he has? You have blessed the work of his hands, so that his flocks and herds are spread throughout the land.

Job 1:10

CHAPTER 3

Steve and I met my freshman year at Mississippi State University, and we married two weeks after I graduated. He was then, and is now more than ever my dearest friend, my closest confidant, and the one true love that every woman prays she will one day find.

We share a lot of similarities and love for many of the same things. But we are as opposite as they come in many ways as well. Call it "genderitis," "introvert vs. extrovert," "husband vs. wife,"—whatever—it doesn't matter. As Forrest Gump says, "We go together like peas and carrots." You can't have one without the other, and in many ways, this is true for Steve and Kristi Brown. We just belong together like a captain and the anchor on the sailboat of life. One sets sail, and the other holds us to the shore.

Our years of marriage have been filled with many moments of laughter, months of heartbreak, hours of tears—both joyful and sad—adventures of travel both near and far, friends who have helped make us who we are today, jobs loved and not so loved, moments of discouragement, and moments of sheer delight in our accomplishments, victories, memories, our times with family, and our blessings.

We have had our share of trials, arguments, and disagreements over the years, but looking back, each emotion that has entered our marriage has been as purposeful to us individually as it has been collectively.

At times, I have struggled somewhat to recount the moments we have shared while writing this book, for many, many of those moments are buried deep in my heart; I do not know that I will ever be able to publicly share all of the more intimate and private things we have lived through. Nor do I believe I am supposed to use this book as a springboard to point out our shortcomings or mistakes like many that are commonly aired today in the media.

Instead, I believe that we should recognize and honor our marriages and relationships as sacred grounds. By doing so, our hearts are safe and our roots are protected so that when the storms come—and they will surely come—we will be able to hunker down and stay planted firmly in the soil that holds us in place and nourishes us from within.

Many of our friends, family, and acquaintances do not understand how or why our marriage is so deeply rooted. We are convinced that Steve was born in the wrong era. If it were up to Steve, he would have lived with, known, and befriended Wyatt Earp. His soul is found in the wild and he will argue anyone that he is closer to the Spirit of God in any hardwood bottom or on any mountaintop than in any other place in this world.

He is rugged and tough enough to hunt and fish and is as efficient at starting a campfire as I am to flipping our thermostat to "heat" when the temperature drops low enough.

Steve is also compassionate, dedicated, and loyal. He is a self-described perfectionist, almost to the point of being obsessive-compulsive, bouncing from one project to the next. It is as if his engine is revved by how much adrenaline he gets going from one project or conversation to the next.

I, on the other hand, am perfectly content for hours on end sitting under an umbrella on the beach, rocking on a porch and marveling at the largeness and serenity of the mountains in North Carolina, or waiting for a storm to roll in. I can outlast any of my friends at a day spa soaking in lagoons or whirlpools, and I love to shop for things that are old, weathered, and shrouded in character. In fact, I seek those same characteristics in my friendships and relationships.

I am purposeful, intentional, creative, and big-picture driven. Steve lives in the moment. I choose to be less spontaneous (although I surprise even myself from time to time) and appreciate a good plan of action.

We both are passionate about our interests, our families, our dogs, and life. We both are closet singers (although I have been known to entertain the shampoo bottles in exchange for a few bubbles). We both love to travel, believe in self-discipline, respect others, and we both love the Lord.

I am the first to admit that we are not perfect. Our marriage is not perfect. But for us, it works, and we're committed to honoring those vows we made on sacred ground so many years ago.

You're probably thinking, *What could be so bad in her life? She's seemingly successful and has a great marriage, a good life...what is it?*

Trust me when I tell you that while we have had our share of awesome memories, as well as some setbacks, nothing could have prepared us for what we would face as heartache, disappointment, and the fight of our lives.

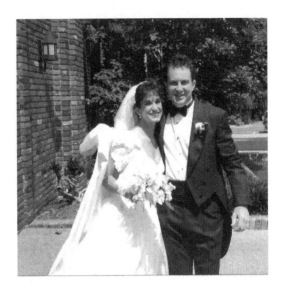

Kristi and Steve—our wedding day—May 31, 1992

So we fix our eyes not on what is seen, but on what is unseen.
For what is seen is temporary but what is unseen is eternal.

2 Corinthians 4:18

CHAPTER 4

In the summer of 1998, after we had been married for six years, Steve and I finally began to feel the tugging toward parenthood. Through the years, well-wishers had teased us that if we were waiting until we were able to afford kids, we'd never have them! That was never our intention, nor did either of us think we had to be secure financially before we started our family.

Granted, there were some things we wanted to do for ourselves, some places we wanted to see, and furniture we wanted to acquire. After all, we had the rest of our lives to be parents. Right?

That's what we were taught. Our generation was nurtured into expectations to wait a little longer to marry and start a family. Careers were the order of the day—sure to provide more opportunities than our families and parents had when they were growing up.

We enjoyed the freedom to leave home for a weekend of camping and white-water rafting, dining with friends, or visiting family without having to consider how to raft with an infant seat or load the car with diapers and Fisher Price® toys!

More important to us, though, and both being from divorced families, we needed to know that we were indeed emotionally ready and equipped to jump from the sidelines into the game of parenting.

Among our friends we had become affectionately known

as the DINKs—double income, no kids. And at church and in the neighborhood, we began to feel quite excluded from the inner circles of afternoon strolls with toddlers in tow, pictures of the little ones with spaghetti draping from their heads, and get-togethers where the topics for discussion centered around whose child was rolling over from side to side and how to make a nursery not smell like a Diaper Genie®.

We were on our *own* timetable—so we told ourselves. Though we were determined not to let peer pressure persuade us into having children just to fit in with others, the tugging continued to manifest slowly and surely.

An annual visit to my gynecologist convinced me it was time to begin trying to get pregnant. Although my sister had been diagnosed several months earlier with premature ovarian failure, my doctor convinced me she believed it was not hereditary, although conceiving could take a little time. After many months—over a year, actually, of being off birth control, I felt deep inside something was wrong. In fact, I *knew* something was wrong.

It wasn't just the fact that month after month, the disappointment came of not conceiving. There were other things I was dealing with. In all that time of being off the birth control pill, I could recall having only one or two monthly cycles. That *couldn't* be normal, I realized.

Additionally, I was moody, irritable, and just downright MEAN. I'd wake up in the night with sweats so bad, I'd strip off all my pajamas and lie on top of the covers only to have to snuggle under them two minutes later. These night sweats were so regular, I became quite proficient at knowing when they were about to hit. One foot hanging out of the sheets helped to balance my temperature, but only if the ceiling fan was at maximum speed!

My neighbors hated me because I was rude and I alienated myself from them. It wasn't on purpose or malicious; I just couldn't get a grip on my thoughts or emotions. Going to the grocery store meant I'd definitely encounter some snotty-nosed kid who didn't know how to bag the groceries just right. And for sure, I thought, *no one* I passed on the road home should have EVER received a license!

And as much as I tried to, I couldn't help the way I was feeling. I couldn't stop my overreactions to things that previously would never have bothered me. I didn't *want* to be that way, did I? Who was this creature from afar that had suddenly inhabited my soul? Had I always been that way? How could I have turned from being named the "friendliest" in school to being this person I didn't even recognize or care to look at in the mirror?

And for Pete's sake, how did *anyone* think I was supposed to get pregnant when the thought of having sex was about as interesting to me as ironing clothes? The drudgery of it left me feeling lonely, tired, and frustrated by my inability to desire it naturally. The physical part of it was just as painful, and it was as if some old, lonely woman who lived in the shoe moved me out of my own body and set up house inside me.

I had no one to talk to about these physical changes. After all, what I was experiencing is so very private that opening up about it—even to family—was out of the question and beyond comprehension. I began to feel like a failure in my marriage. In fact, there were brief moments that I wondered if we would ever make it as a married couple.

One day after a heated argument with Steve, I crouched beside my bed and I remember just wanting the arguments to stop. While it definitely takes two, I had a hard time seeing how my physiological deficiencies could be the root of our frustrations. He begged me to get help, but my stubbornness and pride held out for a while longer.

Recalling these times is like peeling away the layers of an onion. I don't particularly enjoy it, but it is necessary to share and understand what those times added to my life and our marriage. To add to the bitterness, opportunities for us to participate in Mother's Day or Father's Day recognitions at church became so hurtful inside that I began making up excuses to skip church. Surely God would understand. After all, He made me this way, and it was His plan that was keeping us from being able to be a part of all those things. Right?

I rehearsed these types of scenarios for months until I couldn't take it anymore. I was living a life of misery outside of myself and no longer recognized who I was or who I wanted to become. I was pushing everyone away from me without me even realizing it, including my husband. And during those dark months, Satan kept telling me that was so normal. I didn't deserve happiness, he kept telling me. I believed the lies he told me over my shoulder rather than hearing God's whisper in my ear.

Be still and know that I am God;
I will be exalted among the nations, I will be exalted in the earth.

Psalm 46:10

CHAPTER 5

Another annual visit to my gynecologist included some raised eyebrows when I reminded her how long I had been off birth control. She insisted on having some blood drawn and said she would call me with the results.

Several days passed and my anxiety was growing like a balloon sitting on a helium tank nozzle. One more day of waiting, I thought, and I might explode. I called my doctor for answers only to find out that she was out of town. So I left word I was trying to find out the test results. Later that day one of the nurses called me at work.

"Kristi, your test results show you are in menopause," she said. "Were you expecting that?"

The words stormed through my head as I was trying to understand why someone would choose to tell me something so devastating in that way—over the phone and so...matter-of-factly. The force of her words was so strong that I dropped to the floor in my office and had nothing to say. The silence was deafening. My heart felt like someone had ripped it straight from my chest and slung it around like a rag doll being shaken in a pit bull's mouth.

"Ms. Brown, are you there? Would you like the *doctor* to call you?" she sarcastically asked.

"Well, to be honest, I wasn't expecting to hear something like this from a nurse. And, NO, I wasn't expecting to hear this kind of news at all, and I DO want to talk to a doctor!" I exclaimed.

As I hung up the phone, devastation sheared through the very core of me like a tornado whips debris in its path. I ran down the hallway and out the side door of my office building pretending it wasn't happening this way and praying that I would wake up from the nightmare I had suddenly found myself in.

Air. I need air, I thought. I couldn't breathe, and I couldn't stop the tears, even though I still had no idea of how deeply this news would cut into me or what was yet to unfold. A few minutes later, I found myself walking back to my office alone with my news feeling turned upside down and ravaged by the storm within.

Within thirty minutes, one of the other doctors in the clinic whom I had known for a long time called me at work and apologized that the nurse had given me the news in the manner she did. He sounded sympathetic and told me he too was at a loss for words, because he had watched me grow up and knew how hard I must be taking the news.

He referred us to a fertility specialist in Jackson, Mississippi. Within a few days, Steve and I were again headed toward unfamiliar territory. I had cried every tear one person could imagine crying in a lifetime—or so I thought. I was forced to brace myself as best I could for more blood work and consultations that were yet to happen.

Although my new doctor, Dr. John Isaacs, was empathetic and very compassionate toward us, the news came quickly and very hard. Premature ovarian failure was hereditary after all.

It is my understanding that when a woman is tested and monitored for menopause, the numerical range of her FSH (follicle-stimulating hormone), the hormone that determines whether she is in menopause, is somewhere around the fortyish mark. My indicator was over seventy—indicating that not only was I in menopause, but I was on the other end of it. To add to our frustration, Dr. Isaacs confirmed that the only way we would be able to conceive would be through IVF—in vitro fertilization—with an egg donor.

We were handed brochures on IVF and all our other options, including adoption, and it became quite evident that Steve was in denial. I remember hearing him ask about getting a second opinion. Dr. Isaacs just shook his head. He told us we were certainly within our rights to a second opinion, but he felt sure the confirmations and options would be the same.

I didn't see it at the time, but there was my husband, Steve, the family protector, wanting so desperately to find a way to solve this problem for us and find a way to hold on to our dreams that had so quickly slipped through our fingers like dust blowing in the wind.

An hour or so later, I sat holding a prescription for hormone replacement therapy and staring out the car window as we headed for home, with the realization barely soaking in that, just like my sister, I had just been diagnosed with premature ovarian failure at the young age of thirty. We rode home in silence holding hands. But once again, I felt alone in that car and alone in the world. My head hurt, and my heart ached in a way that I had not hurt before. I could hardly even feel I was in the world.

Later that evening, as I laid in the tub, my tears started pouring again. I wept quietly, thinking about the last forty-eight hours or so and how I ended up emotionally in the place I had arrived. The weeping turned to sobs, and I began crying so hard that I barely noticed Steve had come into the bathroom to check on me.

I laid soaking in that tub of warm water, tears streaming

down my face, and my audible cries of anguish beckoned him to come and lift me from the water.

I was too exhausted, too hurt, too parched to even help myself. Mindless and motionless, I stood there as he draped the towel around me and led me to bed—a respite for my body finally drained of the tears.

Oh, if my pillow could speak—a million tears would surely be enough to replace any water that escapes the ocean. And I laid there all night in my own ocean of despair—tossing, turning, and yearning for something solid to believe in or at least a piece of fertile ground to swim toward.

I recounted in my mind over and over the moment, the instant I was told and understood having children on my own would not be an option. My thoughts raced into fast-forward, a glimpse of my life's dreams scurrying ahead of me—seemingly always out of reach. Just always beyond grasp.

There would be no crib to put together, no baby shower, no lullabies, no bouncy seats, or walks with Daddy. Fairies and frogs disappeared from my decorating plans.

I was no stranger to heartache in my life. I learned very early to cope in a world with others' very adult issues. But now this was *my* very adult life and issues. The harsh reality of crushed dreams now belonged to me.

My heart's cry in total exasperation that somehow my body had betrayed me was much too great to bear. "Oh, God, why me?" I asked. "Why are things so hard for me?" How does a thirty-year-old explain to a world of Babies "R" Us and Winnie the Pooh fanatics and those who think they have all the answers that having children is impossible for her?

We're told that we can do or be anything we want. I now had to reconcile that concept with the fact that I could not. Try as I may, I could NEVER have a biological child of my own. I cannot think of anything more devastating to a young wife. We were born to have children, to raise a family, and to leave a legacy behind. Like so many other women, I yearned to wrap those sweet tiny fingers around my own, to smell baby lotion every night, proudly watch my child grow and learn, and to know the depths of my heart from a child's perspective. I wanted to be a mother, but my body could not make it happen. Broken dreams are a part of life, but I wanted more. I wanted to give my husband more than broken dreams. He deserved more.

Plagued by heart-wrenching moments, I replayed friends' innocent comments over and over that night...

"Just relax."

"Stop trying so hard."

"You need to just pray harder."

"It's so much fun practicing though."

"Timing is everything."

Like a bad joke where the punch line falls just short of an audience's acknowledgement, those mindless quips of answers are nothing more than hollow words to a heart broken and an infertile body.

Infertile. Unproductive. Unfruitful. Desolate. That's how I was classified on paper. That's how I felt emotionally. I was barren.

Jesus turned and said to them, "Daughters of Jerusalem, do not weep for me; weep for yourselves and for your children. For the time will come when you will say, 'Blessed are the barren women, the wombs that never bore and the breasts that never nursed!'

Luke 23:28-29

CHAPTER 6

It took less than a month of taking hormones to feel a significant difference in myself. I had forgotten what it was like to laugh. I had not realized how lethargic I had become. And the night sweats and hot flashes were more under control than ever. I even smiled at the kids who bagged my groceries.

As contradictory as it may seem, a big part of me became relieved about my diagnosis. At least now I had confirmation, medical evidence, and a reason that I wasn't losing my mind; the symptoms I had been experiencing were indeed symptoms of a bigger problem than I could've imagined having to face at thirty—menopause. And I finally realized—the months of not recognizing myself was not my fault.

By summer, I felt triumphant on some days because I was starting to see semblances of the person I had known once upon a time. I slowly became interested in my life and others' lives again. It was not a moment too soon, as I needed to mend some bridges that had begun a slow descent into the torrential waters of life. My marriage was not in danger of drifting away, but the unexplainable moods and lack of intimacy kept Steve and me at odds more than we cared to mention or I dared to acknowledge.

We began looking for a new home—a change of scenery, we thought, would help heal the wounds. We finally settled on a home six miles out of town with over five acres of hardwoods and a view of deer that have become an annual ritual to watch from the kitchen at the first feel of an autumn breeze.

The house needed some updated paint and décor, and I jumped in with vigor—picking out colors for every room. I was up for the task and it gave me something to believe in and dream about, and it was a welcome break to see tangible results.

But those who hope in the LORD will renew their strength. They will soar on wings like eagles; they will run and not grow weary, they will walk and not be faint.

Isaiah 40:31

CHAPTER 7

A few months after moving into our new home, the longing for a dog started to fill my heart and mind. I am sure Steve thought I had reverted into a five-year-old begging for her first pet. I wanted a yellow Lab. Period. He talked to breeders and friends of breeders looking for the right one from which we would purchase a furry ball of frolicking fun. And when the call came one evening from Poplar Ridge Retrievers that a litter of pups would be born in about six weeks, I could hardly contain myself. That's all I talked about. Puppy this, puppy that. The day would not come soon enough.

It was early springtime by then, and my grandmother was going into the hospital for heart surgery. My mother flew in from Houston, Texas, to be in Oxford, Mississippi, for the surgery, and I promised to meet my family at the hospital as soon as I could leave work a little early that day.

I made it to the hospital after Grandmom had gone into surgery, and I waited with the family laughing and enjoying being surrounded by those who loved me most. I was looking forward to seeing her sit up in bed and giggle when she realized I had come to visit.

Our family was called into a different room to wait for the surgeon. We were expecting to be briefed on a successful procedure, but the minute the surgeon entered the room, I knew. Grandmom was gone.

I felt sick to my stomach and had that urge to run again.

I looked around at my family in disbelief that our family matriarch was no longer with us, and I realized I had not been there to see that final twinkle in her eye prior to surgery.

I sat there on the floor crying and thinking about the hippity hop ball I used to bounce on under her feet. I could taste the fried chocolate pies and the homemade chicken potpies she would make especially for me when I'd come to visit. She had a way of making each of her grandchildren feel they were the most special of all. I thought of the shame-shames (fern-like plants that we named when we were small. We named them while lightly rubbing the leaves and singing "shame, shame on you..." while their leaves delicately closed up), and the muscadines and daylilies on the hillside needed her still. I needed her still.

She taught me to can green beans and to build frog houses in the sandbox. She'd give me free access to her Tupperware to play with in that sandbox, and I suddenly had the urge to go to her house and hide under the dining room table draped in the blue sheets we used to build a fort under. Her giggle was contagious, and I miss her terribly—even today.

Grandmom was to be buried in her family's plot in Booneville, Mississippi. The day we drove through downtown Booneville to her graveside services, I looked up and saw the store where she worked one time. *Sadie's.* I remembered hearing stories of times past and knew she had fun memories of working there at that five-and-dime store. The name struck me, though, with that feeling we all get from time to time when we know something is meant to be.

It occurred to me that "Sadie" was such a Southern name and my female Lab yet to be born would be named Sadie. It was a gift and a special bond with my Grandmom that I couldn't explain—not even to myself. On the way home, I stopped at a pet store and bought Sadie a purple collar with hand-painted daisies on it. She would have to grow quite a bit before she would fit into it, but my Grandmom's love for flowers, dogs, and *Sadie's* took on a whole new meaning for me that day.

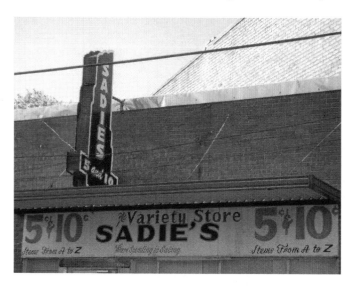

Sadie's in Booneville, Mississippi

CHAPTER 8

A month later, on April 13, we received a call that the pups had been born. I waited two weeks and drove by myself to Blue Springs, just north of Tupelo, Mississippi, to see them. I was drawn instantly to the lightest-colored pup that was in the corner of the box. While the rest of the puppies were scootin' around, she was sleeping peacefully. I picked her up, nestled her to my ear, and I knew she was mine. She grunted a few of those wonderful little puppy grunts while I held her close. I spoke to her, called her by name, and vowed to protect her and love her always.

Two and a half weeks later, I was back again, visiting my Sadie, and this time, her eyes were open and she was much fatter than the first time we met. That little roly-poly white, furry ball followed me around the breeder's yard until she couldn't do it anymore, and I was convinced she not only knew who I was but she also knew her name. Her ears would perk up whenever I called her. I was in love with this puppy, and could hardly wait the remaining two to three weeks before we could bring her home.

We finally brought her home, and Sadie fell in love with being loved. Our five acres were a Lab's wonderland, and, over the next few weeks, we watched Sadie blossom into the sassiest little thing.

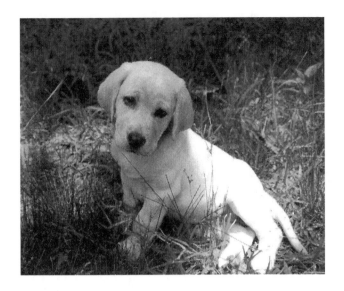

Sadie's first week home with us - June 2001

Every afternoon she helped us pick up sticks. She chased off deer early in the mornings, and learned what it felt like to saturate herself completely in the mud hole in our driveway.

Sadie filled a void for me at a time when I needed a diversion the most. We snuggled on the sofa every night and played hard every day. Everywhere we went, she went too and drew a lot of attention. She acclimated into our lives extremely well and to this day, she has never destroyed a single thing we own. Faithful Sadie—ever the protector, loving dog, and dearest companion. My heart has always been safe with Sadie nearby.

About fifteen months after we brought Sadie home, Lily entered our lives, and our home has never been the same since. Lily was one of twelve puppies born from a friend's male yellow Lab and his across-the-street companion's litter. Lily is, well, as one could imagine, almost lily-white—a very feminine description for the tomboy dog that she is. Lock, stock, and barrel, Lily came in and rocked our worlds, demanding attention that she couldn't have possibly gotten from her littermates. She is as athletic as dogs come and requires a lot of exercise and head pats.

It took several weeks for Sadie to realize that, although she was aptly named and registered as Princess Sadie Brown, she would have to share her throne with Lily, the rambunctious dog!

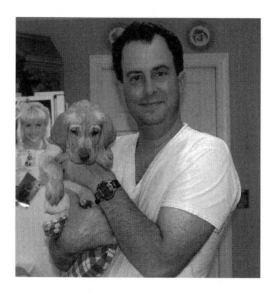

Steve holding Lily after her first bath.

During that same year, Steve and I had saved and planned a two-week trip to New Zealand in honor of our tenth-year wedding anniversary. We got married in May, but the trip was planned for October. Seasons are opposite from the United

States, so an October trip meant an early spring in New Zealand and Steve would be able to hunt turkeys over there!

I guess I'm a sucker for punishment because we turkey hunted the first few days of our two-week vacation. Imagine my delight, though, when I was the first of us to harvest a New Zealand bird. I'm not sure if that has ever been admitted publicly. For goodness sakes, it needs to be known!

By the time we returned from our grand adventure, Sadie and Lily had become fast friends and had learned how to play, eat, and sleep together as the Brown girls. I almost didn't recognize Lily because she grew so much just in those two weeks we were gone. But I was especially touched that our dog sitter kept a diary of their daily activities and frolics, so that I was able to have a glimpse into their "doggie-day-care" musings. Anyone who is endeared to animals, especially dogs, would understand how my maternal instinct was at its peak over those precious dogs.

How great is the love the Father has lavished upon us that we might be called children of God.

1 John 3:1

CHAPTER 9

Mid-October 2002

For months on end, we intentionally did not make any decisions about our family. When we first learned about my infertility, we took time to grieve and decided it was best to not hurry into a choice.

A couple of weeks before our trip to New Zealand, we were sitting in our den and before either of us realized it, our conversation turned into the decision to begin exploring our IVF option. I was stunned; I just sat there knowing I needed to pick my jaw up off the floor. Were we actually ready again to dream this dream?

Later that night I realized it had taken us nearly three years to come to peace with the decision of exploring IVF. It wasn't something we had talked about much over the past few years because we both had definite convictions about the procedure.

It was extremely important to us that whatever decision we made about having children, either through IVF or adoption, it would be because we truly wanted a child, not just because we couldn't naturally have a baby. I am not sure if that statement resonates with you, the reader. I have known many people who have gotten caught up in the "not being able to have a baby," that they are in the whirlwind of "Oh, let's do this, or let's try this" simply to prove that they can. I felt very strongly that I needed to know, without a shadow of a doubt, we really wanted a baby for us.

The next day I made an excited phone call to Dr. Isaacs' office in search of specifics on what we needed to do to pursue anonymous egg donation. Days later, the paperwork came, and as we sat down to review it, we both became more and more excited about the possibilities.

We listed all of our personal medical information and all the requirements we wished for in someone willing to donate an egg. It was a precious opportunity to put down on paper what was important to us. But at the end of the day, we knew that most of the qualities on the list did not matter. Successfully fulfilling our hopes and dreams for a healthy baby was all we really wanted.

Once we submitted our paperwork, it took only a few months to be matched. In fact, the phone call came sooner than I anticipated. As the nurse poured out specific details about the background of this donor, I began to cry. Many of our requirements on the wish list were addressed in some way. And I knew then, a connection was there; a purpose was unfolding. We accepted the donor and pursued the medical details with insurance and doctors visits.

The next few months required multiple visits to the doctor's office and multiple visits for our donor to the office, as well. I became what my husband referred to as a human pincushion. Medicines were ordered and sent via mail to our house, and I had to learn to inject myself with shots for weeks and weeks in preparation for "the big day." I wondered every day about our donor—how she was feeling, if she was doing similar things to her body, if she was taking care of herself.

Finally, the day came and it was our chance to hopefully have an embryo implanted. That July, we were all set for the transfer. It was quite an exciting time, and I could hardly think of anything else. Steve and I continuously talked about the exciting "what ifs" and "we'll never say this or that to our child" dialogues. We smiled at each other a lot during the preparation times, each knowing that whatever happened would surely change us forever. I was required to go down to Jackson the Sunday before to have my uterus measured to make sure the hormone injections had indeed been working.

I wish I could write a happily-ever-after ending here and that we were given the thumbs-up right away, but, true to form for my body, my uterus lining was at the minimum amount of measured thickness allowable to make the transfer. After all the weeks and weeks of injections, I was shocked, quite frankly, that the hormone injections yielded such a minimal result. Dr. Isaacs was just as surprised. I never dreamed that we would have a setback such as that, but, after talking through what it all meant, Dr. Isaacs was comfortable knowing I still had a few more injections over the next couple of days. The decision was made to push forward with the plan.

He replied, "Because you have so little faith. I tell you the truth,
if you have faith as small as a mustard seed, you can say to this
mountain, 'Move from here to there' and it will move. Nothing will
be impossible for you."

Matthew 17:20

CHAPTER 10

Our anonymous egg donor was scheduled for egg retrieval a couple of days before the intended transfer. I was at work when the nurse called to let me know we had an outstanding harvest with twenty-one eggs retrieved. Clinically, the next step was to put the eggs and Steve's sperm together for fertilization early that morning. Statistics showed and we had every reason to believe and hope that we could potentially have fourteen to seventeen fertilized eggs for not only this implantation, but future opportunities as well. We were very excited and confident about the success rate.

By late afternoon I received another call. Our nurse's voice had a tone of disbelief when she identified herself on the phone. I was a little anxious about that as my heart sunk. She explained to me that as it turned out, of the twenty-one harvested eggs, only one little egg fertilized on its own.

I sat there—alone—again with the news that I felt was almost a deal breaker for continuing on this journey. Could we continue forward with the procedure? What does that mean? Of all the things we had been through, I couldn't help but think of that one little fertilized egg saying, "Ta-da!! I made it!"

In fact, in a split moment that felt like a half hour, I had visions of that fertilized egg three years down the road. "She" had brown curly hair and giggled at ladybugs and daffodils while twirling in our yard in a play dress, saying, "Ta-da...Ta-da!" I could see her smiling at me.

The nurse told me of another step they would be taking to try to inject the eggs directly with the sperm. The technical term doesn't matter, but I knew we had come too far to just quit. I called Steve to let him know the seesaw news. Our family's future teetered on whether or not the procedure would yield more opportunities to have more than one egg implanted in me. We waited overnight for the news.

Another phone call confirmed that through the in-lab technology, three more little eggs were fertilized the following day, giving us the chance for at least one out of the four.

The day of implantation came and Dr. Isaacs suggested we implant all four fertilized eggs in me. I was scared to death. *Four eggs?* I thought. What would we do with more than one? Somehow I knew in the back of my mind that multiples are always a big part of in vitro, but would we really be ready? Steve held my hand the entire way through the procedure, and I knew we would be OK.

Some women just know the instant they get pregnant. Thirty minutes later, I knew.

I was sent home with a picture of the fertilized eggs prior to implantation and they were beautiful. I framed the photo and carried it with me everywhere I went. To this day, it is one of the most fascinating photos I have ever seen.

I had felt a connection to the first egg and was more than thrilled to learn a week later that I was indeed pregnant. My HCG levels were off the charts within that first week, which we learned could be an indicator for a multiples pregnancy. My heart was soaring for the first time in a very long time, and I felt great.

The following few weeks were filled with sheer excitement, premature shopping, and planning for what would surely change our lives and bring us the joy of family we so desired and longed to have.

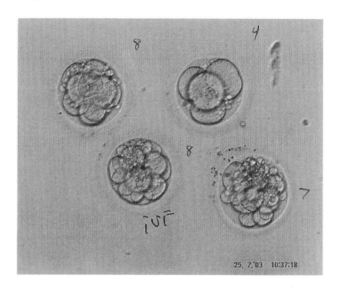

Where "life" all began, July 2003.

CHAPTER 11

Around week nine of my pregnancy, I began to get sick, which I thought was simply morning sickness. At first I did not complain about the sickness. After all, I felt it was a small sacrifice and part of the process of being pregnant. I learned very early to rationalize this.

I stocked up on crackers and milk. Mashed potatoes became my daily lunch menu. I had such an insatiable appetite for vegetables that I am sure I drank a grocery store full of V-8® juice in a week's time. Although I had never been a tomato juice fan, I couldn't get enough of it.

Around the tenth week, my sickness began to worsen for me physically. As the nausea and sickness continued, I was unable to keep anything in and the frequency of my vomiting increased. I began waking up in the middle of the night and falling asleep hovered over the toilet just so I could already be there the next time the urge came.

Stress at work during that time was almost too much for me. And while I knew my pregnancy sickness was not the result of the stress I was experiencing in the workplace, I could tell my blood pressure was elevating daily while I was at work. I had never had blood pressure problems, but I just knew something was off. I was gaining weight almost daily, it seemed. At one point, I thought I was imagining things until I realized one day my ankles were swelling.

"Is this normal?" I asked Teresa, a good friend with

whom I worked. She took one look at me and insisted I call my doctor.

I am positive I sounded like a pregnant first timer with the concerns I voiced over the phone that day. However, I convinced the nurse on the phone that I needed to come in when I told her about my swelling. She told me to come in that afternoon. Although I am usually self-sufficient and independent enough to take myself to the doctor, Teresa offered to drive me that day. Inside I was very relieved because deep down, I felt like I needed someone to be with me. I was already shaky and nervous from my elevated blood pressure, and I just needed a friend. At that instant in our friendship, there was nothing more to be said. Woman to woman—she knew without my asking what I needed.

I later learned she was reprimanded at work for taking time to be with me. In fact, she was told it wasn't part of her job description. There are just some people in this world who cannot comprehend what it means to be true to oneself and to put others' needs before their own. And self-absorbed attitudes, especially among people who are personally and/or professionally insecure, are a desperate attempt by Satan himself to create doubt, hurt, and confusion. These people are weeds in our life's gardens.

Nonetheless, I will be forever indebted to Teresa; she is, most definitely, a friend everyone would hope to have and to be.

A man of many companions may come to ruin, but there is a friend who sticks closer than a brother.

Proverbs 18:24

CHAPTER 12

The nurse greeted me almost instantly when I arrived and took me back to triage for the standard blood pressure and temperature checks and a weigh-in. When she weighed me, I had gained nine pounds in less than three weeks since my first visit to their office. This was something so contrary to the fact that I had been so sick. She was baffled and commented that most people would've probably lost weight.

I could see a look of confusion and compassion in her eyes as she walked me to the examination room. There I waited alone for my OB/GYN to come and assure me I would be fine. I reasoned it all out and convinced myself that I would probably be put on bed rest since this was considered a higher-risk pregnancy.

My doctor came in and decided to do an ultrasound that day. As he rolled the cold instrument over my abdomen and took computerized pictures of the baby, he began asking me if I had ever been told about "molar pregnancies" since I was a fertility patient. Instantly, I felt like someone had left out a key piece of information I needed to know, so I told him I had no idea what he was talking about. I had never even heard of a *molar pregnancy*.

Then it came. Like a loud thud off in the distance, I wasn't sure of the source, only that I heard it. "Get dressed and meet me in my office. We'll talk there. Do you have someone with you today?"

"Yes, my friend is in the waiting room," I replied. And with my answer the door closed quietly and he disappeared.

Why did he just ask that? I thought. *Wonder why he can't just talk to me here and send me on my way?* My mind began swirling as I got dressed. I felt light-headed and weak but my curiosity and adrenalin began pumping so quickly that I dressed and began looking for his office as fast as I could. I was beginning to shake from aroused nerves.

I rounded the corner to his office, and Teresa was waiting for me there. "How are you feeling?" she asked.

"Not sure. I don't know what's happening," I replied nervously while I searched my friend's eyes for any assurance that I would be fine.

She grabbed my hand when my doctor entered the room. There it was again. Thud. Another bomb being dropped.

My doctor began explaining to us that my pregnancy was what he felt was a "molar pregnancy."

"A what?" I asked. I explained I had never heard of such a thing and no one had ever explained it to me. So he patiently tried to describe what would become a very puzzling and complicated situation for me.

In simple terms, there are two types of molar pregnancies. One involves a growth in the placenta that masks itself as a pregnancy, but does not have an embryo at all. The second type does involve a baby, yet abnormal cells (cancerous) begin to develop in the placenta, causing the placenta to grow exponentially. My molar pregnancy indeed involved a baby. In my case, at twelve weeks pregnant, my body and placenta were measuring the same size as a healthy eighteen-week pregnancy. That definitely explained the weight gain.

My OB/GYN continued to explain that a molar pregnancy also means the baby would have three sets of chromosomes, which is incompatible with life. He humbly explained in cases like mine there would be no way I could carry the baby to term and expect to have a healthy baby. He scheduled an emergency meeting for the very next day with a fetal specialist, who happened to be in the same group as my fertility specialist in Jackson, Mississippi.

I don't even remember leaving his office but I remember having to call Steve, who was working two and a half hours away from home that day. I didn't know how to tell him— over a cell phone—the crushing news I had just received. So I simply told him he needed to come home immediately and that we were being referred to a fetal specialist the very next morning. Teresa, who had been with me the entire day, took me home and stayed with me. She held and comforted me until Steve arrived.

Though you have made me see troubles, many and bitter, you will restore my life again...
My lips will shout for joy when I sing praise to you.

Psalms 71:20, 23

CHAPTER 13

We decided together to call our parents and I knew I had to dig deeper than I knew how to and put on a brave face and voice. "It was just preventative" was how we described the necessary appointment with promises to call the next day once we knew more.

That night I felt like I had just a couple of years earlier as I laid in the bathtub the night I had learned that, indeed, I was infertile. Alone and barren.

I threw up off and on until I went to bed that night, and I was sure it was partly because I had cried so much. Frighteningly though, my vomiting and sickness peaked that night in a way I had never experienced. Finding words to convey how seriously sick I was, is more than difficult.

Steve and I were up the entire night because, literally, every half hour I was vomiting. Crackers and Gatorade® wouldn't even stay down. Steve put a deep pan in the bed with us because I became so weak I could no longer roll out of bed to make it to the bathroom.

At one point, the vomiting was so severe and violent, that I was on my knees, holding on to the headboard, throwing up into the pan where my pillow should have been. It was the worst feeling physically I had ever had or have had since. In fact, it was so impactful that it became a measurement for me for what I would come to face in the very near future.

When daylight rose, Steve helped me dress. Even as gross

as I felt, I had no strength for a shower, and was hardly able to pull a brush through my hair. I could barely brush my teeth, because it made me gag and I was just so physically worn out from being sick.

Still, I threw up the entire way to Jackson and once we settled into the waiting room in the doctor's office, I laid across Steve's lap because holding my head up took energy I no longer had.

We were soon ushered into a room of high-powered medical computers and monitors that were on several walls surrounding the examination table. As I had done so many times during this whole procedure, I undressed and laid down for yet another ultrasound. And there "she" was. Very low on my pelvic bone, I felt the instrument rubbing back and forth until "her" silhouette became so obviously clear. I saw her toes, her thumb, her head. I held Steve's hand as we watched the monitors. Tears streamed down my cheeks.

For a few moments, our hearts soared at seeing the life growing inside me. But the stark realization and complete disbelief that what we were seeing was something that humanly could not exist as it developed was more than my heart could bear. The placenta resembled what the specialist referred to as a "Swiss cheese" effect—an image with varying sizes of holes.

Additionally, we were given the heart-wrenching news that we must terminate the pregnancy in order to save my life. The baby would never have survived, and I would continue to get sicker if we didn't.

The specialist and nurse left us alone for a few moments to be by ourselves as we absorbed the worst news we ever wanted to hear. I cried. Steve cried. It was as if what we were seeing on the monitors was a sick lie. How could that precious image be "incompatible" with life? How could this horrible thing be happening to us? I turned away from the monitors and just laid there with tears still streaming down my cheeks. Amazingly, I managed to make it through those few moments without getting sick.

The specialist came back in and, while he was talking, the images disappeared off the monitors. Gone forever from view, but delicately framed in my mind and heart, our baby became a part of my life's secret museum, which I visit from time to time.

I felt like my hopes and dreams had been stripped down to medical words that rang through the hollow halls of my heart. The part of the earth I walked on was once again barren, lifeless, and unfruitful. I somehow felt I had failed— again—and that I had disappointed those closest to me—most importantly my husband.

He deserved a family of his own. He deserved more than I could give him or ever would be able to give him. He deserved happiness, not despair, and I felt like I offered him nothing but a series of disappointment after disappointment.

Know also that wisdom is sweet to your soul; if you find it, there is a future hope for you, and your hope will not be cut off."

Proverbs 24:14

CHAPTER 14

Once I redressed, we were taken to another consult room and in walked another doctor. He introduced himself as Dr. Jimmy Moore, a gynecological oncologist, and immediately offered his condolences for what we were experiencing. Looking back on this moment, I barely remember meeting him. At the time, he was just another physician to get us through this nightmare. I just remember him explaining a little more in depth as to why we found ourselves meeting with an oncologist. Something about how he would be a part of the "procedure." And while they were fairly certain I had a molar pregnancy, there were still some things unanswered. They were still waiting for a final HCG count from my blood work, which would help finalize their diagnosis. Terms like evacuation, molar cells, and subsequent follow-ups swirled around the conference room. I remember hearing him say in 80 percent of similar cases, no further action would be necessary and that we had every reason to believe I would be fine. In many cases, women with molar pregnancies go on to have future healthy pregnancies.

He disappeared momentarily and returned with admission orders for the hospital that adjoined their offices. I found myself being taken by wheelchair through a maze of empty hallways while Steve moved our car to the hospital parking lot.

I was admitted right away and put in a private room on the maternity floor. As I was wheeled down the hall, door after door greeted me with either pale pink or sky blue wreaths, ribbons, and flowers.

By the time Steve found me, I already had an IV of fluids started in me because I was so dehydrated and needed some relief from the nausea and vomiting.

Steve called my mom and his parents and began the long list of calls to friends who were concerned and needed to know what was happening.

While we waited for familial support to arrive, Steve and I shared some time, just the two of us. I told him I just wanted it to be over, and that I didn't think I could go through this again. I knew what was happening all around me and what it meant to finally utter those words. My head knew I had to say good-bye to my heart's desire, but my heart was breaking into so many pieces that I did not know if I would ever be able to gather them up again.

Later that evening my mother arrived, and I cried the moment I saw her. The heartache of not giving her a grandchild was impossibly crippling. I wanted to tell her everything would be alright, but I had not gotten to that point yet myself. I searched her eyes for strength. I knew I would never know what she must have been feeling for her youngest daughter. My life or my heart would never be able to relate to hers in a maternal way.

Steve's parents came in a little later and I am sure he was as grateful to have them there as I was to have my mother with me. Their love, prayers, support, and strength helped us dig a little deeper to face the next morning's procedure.

I was given plenty of fluids intravenously through the night as well as anti-anxiety and nausea medications. I dozed in and out while my family gathered around me using my hospital bed as a makeshift picnic blanket complete with a dinner of Subway® sandwiches. I was not hungry nor was I allowed much more than clear liquids at this point, anyway. I remember them circling my bed before visiting hours were over, holding hands, and praying for the next day. I remember thinking even in my grogginess that tomorrow's sun would rise on the rest of the world but hard rains and storms were definitely in our forecast. Darkness loomed in the room and in my heart.

*When we walk to the edge of all the light
we have and take that step into the darkness
of the unknown, we must believe that one
of two things will happen—there will be
something solid for us to stand on, or
God will teach us how to fly.*

-Patrick Overton

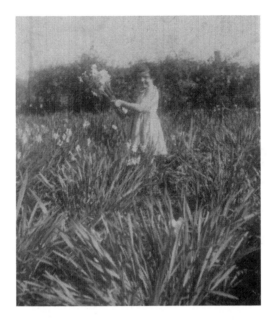

My mother as a young girl gathering daffodils.

CHAPTER 15

On October 2, our hearts shattered as we sent our baby to be with the Lord. I was taken very early for my D and C, a procedure used to evacuate the uterus. Physically, mentally, emotionally, I was exhausted. My mood was somber while I was being rolled down that long hallway of doors decorated in pinks and blues. I closed my eyes and just prayed for it to be over. I don't remember anything until I saw Dr. Moore standing over me in the operating room. I had been given some medication already and was very relaxed as he spoke to me. He and Dr. Perry, the fetal specialist, promised to take care of me, and I closed my teary eyes and drifted off to sleep.

I woke up with the subliminal knowledge that I was on a gurney in the middle of a hallway at the hospital. I could hear the nurses talking about me and trying to wake me up. All I wanted to do was sleep—but first,

"I think I'm going to be sick!" I exclaimed as I barely rolled to the side of my bed and vomited. I've always had a low tolerance for anesthesia.

I heard one nurse say, "I don't know why they did this up here—it's too much..."

I later understood what she meant, but all I could think of was, "God, save me. Please, God, make this stop."

I woke up again with the realization that I was in a completely different room and I was alone. *It must be over,* I thought. *It's over. I'm different now and my baby is gone.*

Where is everyone? I wondered, as I pried my eyes open to see that I had been put into a birth suite for delivering mothers.

Tears rolled out the corners of my eyes, and I felt miserable. I needed to go to the bathroom but knew it would be out of the question for me to get up. I looked over at the IV stand and realized I was being given blood. No wonder I was so hot. The combination of fluids elevated my body temperature and as I began to ask for help, the nurse came in to check on me.

She told me they would be taking me back to my room once they finished giving me blood. I had obviously lost a lot during the "procedure." I was weak and didn't really care anyway.

The room was large; the television was on, yet I began to hear voices that were more recognizable to me. My family was nearby, and I began to feel a little calmer. My sister walked in the room followed by my mother, and it was another one of those woman-to-woman moments that I will never forget. They walked over to me, around the IV stand and monitors, and managed to hug me and give me that "knowing" look that we women understand. Their eyes searched mine for any emotion I might be feeling and I managed to smile a little.

"How are you?" I asked my sister, Lori.

"I'm good and am so glad to see you," she said.

"Where's Steve?" I asked.

"He went with his parents to get something to eat."

"OK." I sighed.

A bit later I was rolled back down the pink and blue decorated hallway to my room and noticed a sticker of a white dove on my door.

Steve was there, along with my family, as the nurses got me settled. The room was already filling up with plants and floral arrangements and notes from our friends.

I dozed in and out for a while until we received a special visitor. A nurse came in and brought a special box to me. She explained that because we were on the maternity floor, the white dove on the door was a way to let all the caregivers know that we had lost our baby. Additionally, the box she gave us included some inspirational tracts, a small white Bible, and a silver heart charm. She also let us know that if at any time, I was "uncomfortable" on that floor, they would make arrangements to move us. I was touched by their awareness of my feelings and emotions but assured her I would be fine. I would probably be going home the next day anyway, I thought.

Dr. Moore dropped by and introduced me to Beth, his nurse. She was a petite young woman with the warmest eyes. She stood at the end of my bed looking at me and I realized as Dr. Moore was talking, her eyes began to tear up. She felt like a kindred spirit, although I had never met her before.

Dr. Moore told me that prior to the D and C they had been waiting for my HCG hormone calculations from the previous day. He informed us that I had been a very sick woman. According to the number of weeks of my pregnancy, my levels should have ranged anywhere from 14,000 to 140,000. It took a very long time to get a reading on mine, but when they finally got the calculation at 750,000, the molar pregnancy was confirmed.

I was stunned—speechless actually. It was so much to take in, yet I knew all along that something had not been right. And we did what we had to do—there was no other choice in the matter. At that time, my head was much more in control than my heart.

I sent my mom and sister to the hotel for the night and worked on eating whatever bland meal had been brought to the room. Several of our friends in the area came by to visit, and I did my best to put on a brave face as they searched for words of sympathy and support for us. I felt so sorry for them because I knew they wouldn't know what to say. It was at that moment in time I learned that it doesn't matter what you say to someone going through a sorrowful time, just let them know you care. The fact that they took time out of their lives and schedules to just show up for us was very touching for me. It was reassuring to know we had friends who cared so much for us.

The next day, Mom and Lori arrived very early to see me, and we decided they would drive back to Starkville to get my house cleaned up in expectation that I would probably get to go home later that day or the next. I was thankful for their visit but was also grateful for some time alone and to be with Steve. But as the day progressed, I regressed. I was having trouble feeling like I was getting enough air and started a dry, hacking cough.

Someone ordered breathing treatments for me and I was given that little tube up my nose for oxygen. I hated that nose piece but it gave me a little relief.

Through the night, I woke up off and on and realized I was having trouble raising myself up. My back was hurting just below my shoulder blades. And suddenly there it was...off in the distance, I heard the sound of a baby crying. I lay there thinking, *God, I cannot do this. It is not fair.* Tears flooded my pillow and I rolled myself over to face the wall for the rest of the night.

The next morning I complained so much about my inability to breathe that they finally decided to take X-rays, which ended up showing that I had an abundance of fluid on my lungs from all the fluids I had been given upon admission as well as the blood transfusion.

Instead of getting to go home, I was kept another day and put on a catheter so that I could have a Lasix treatment to pull the fluid off my lungs.

Hour after hour, the fluid emptied and I wondered if it would ever end. I was ready to get out of there. I had been there since Wednesday and it was already Saturday. Four days was long enough. And the crying babies were a constant reminder of that white dove on my door.

Finally, I was released on Sunday and we arrived home to find my mother and sister had not only cleaned our house, but had decorated for fall with a couple of small hay bales and potted mums arranged on our patio area just beyond my French doors for me to enjoy.

Bless them. I had been so sick in the previous weeks that cleaning house had not been my priority nor was decorating for fall. They knew this and just as women do, especially in my family, they wanted me to come home to fresh linens, a clean toilet, food in the fridge, and something pretty to look at!

...Open wide your mouth and I will fill it.

Psalms 81:10

CHAPTER 16

As I began to heal emotionally and physically over the next couple of weeks, I remained under Dr. Moore's watchful eye as he followed my HCG levels down. I was given strict orders to have my blood drawn weekly to check my hormone levels; as long as they were dropping, I would probably never hear from him.

I drove to Columbus (a city located approximately thirty minutes east from my hometown) once a week for three weeks to have my blood work drawn. Each week, the lab faxed the results to Dr. Moore in Jackson. Each day I was feeling physically stronger. I was still taking sick leave from work and was thankful for it because I was finally beginning to go through the grieving process. Day after day, cards, letters and bouquets of flowers arrived, and I was in awe of how many people took the time to let me know they were thinking of us.

One particular Wednesday morning I had been enjoying some quiet time on my patio reading and praying. I had not been in the habit of a quiet time on a regular basis, but my life was different now. My heart was different, and I felt it was the most important thing I could ever do. It was a beautiful fall day, and I'll never forget the way the sun glimmered through our woods. Golden leaves were trickling down onto our tree-covered yard. The air was clean and crisp, and it had been such a long time since I had really taken the time to capture a fall day in the album of my heart. I was intent on going back to work the following week and had just spoken with my friend and colleague, Teresa, to let her know I would be back that following Monday.

I was listening to a Ginny Owens CD she had given me, and a song came on that encouraged me and spoke to me to have peace. As the CD played, I wrote the words to that song in my journal.

Every verse of that song, every word, and every note resonated through me that the Lord had work for me. That instant, as I was praying and writing in my journal, a peace flooded my soul in a way that I cannot explain. Sometimes there are no words adequate to share what is happening in one's life. As I wrote, I looked up at that big blue fall sky and felt a surge of joy enter my heart. I totally gave my desire to have a baby over to the Lord. It's in black and white in my journal entry that day. I sat there and read the words over and over. There's no way that I could have been strong enough on my own to turn that desire over. It was from the Holy Spirit. And with a joy that few people really can know, I was finally ready to give Him complete control in my life and to use me however, wherever, whenever He was ready. It was a pivotal moment in my life and one that is as fresh and sweet to me today as it was when it happened. I was in the valley and He led me there for a purpose, and I agreed to walk in it.

If You Want Me To (by Ginny Owens/Kyle Matthews)*

The pathway is broken
And the signs are unclear
And I don't know the reason why You brought me here
But just because You love me the way that You do
I'm gonna walk through the valley

If You want me to

No I'm not who I was
When I took my first step
And I'm clinging to the promise You're not through with me
yet
So if all of these trials bring me closer to You
Then I will go through the fire
If You want me to

It may not be the way I would have chosen
When You lead me through a world that's not my home
But You never said it would be easy
You only said I'll never go alone

So when the whole world turns against me
And I'm all by myself
And I can't hear You answer my cries for help
I'll remember the suffering Your love put You through
And I will walk through the valley
If You want me to

As I was finishing up my three-hour morning with my time of reflection that day, my phone was ringing. It was Dr. Moore, the oncologist from Jackson.

"Kristi, do you remember me telling you that as long as your HCG levels were dropping you'd never hear from me?"

"Yes," I hesitantly answered.

"Well, I've been charting your levels over the past few weeks. You'll recall we started out at 750,000 and last week we saw them fall to 62,000," he said.

"Yes, I know."

"This week they've risen back up to 250,000, which leads me to believe those molar cells have probably metastasized."

I sat there listening very closely to what he was telling me. I started shivering and I realized I was alone again—with this news.

"So what happens now?" I bravely asked—afraid of what he would say.

"I've already scheduled a CT scan for tomorrow here in Jackson. We don't need to wait any longer. Come to our offices but pack an overnight bag."

I called Steve, my mother, and Teresa to let them all know the latest news. Mom made plans to come down that evening and travel with us the next day.

I sat down at my dining room table with my journal open to the day's entry and realized that, at *that* moment, I had to *mean* what I had just prayed and written. The realization hit me so hard—I had turned it all over to God, and He literally took me at my word. I learned He was not finished with that part of the tilling process in my journey.

CHAPTER 17

We traveled to Jackson, and I tried to prepare myself mentally for the CT scan. I was given a thick, chalky white mixture to drink, and I barely made it to the trash can in the waiting room before it all came back up. I sat on the floor with white foam pouring from my mouth. I was humiliated in front of the strangers in the waiting room, and I sat there and cried. The staff scurried to my side and helped me clean up before giving me instructions to just go on over to the radiologist's office. I would get to drink something more like "lemonade" when I arrived. It tasted more like arsenic lemonade, but it stayed down. I prayed it would stay down because the sooner I was able to be scanned, the sooner I would know the results. Neither my body nor my mind could handle another nauseous moment.

I was finally able to have the scan and I took the films back to Dr. Moore's office for him to look at them. When we got outside, Steve and I pulled them out of the envelope, and though I wasn't quite sure what we were looking at, I saw what looked like holes in my lungs. Indeed, the CT scan confirmed our greatest fear—the "mole" cells from the pregnancy had indeed metastasized to my lungs, liver, and uterus.

I was furious. When the news officially came from Dr. Moore, I remember being in a private consult room in his office, and I wanted to start slinging the neatly lined up books off the bookshelves. I was that angry and I wanted everybody to know it. It was not fair! My reaction completely caught me off guard.

OK, God. What are you doing? I thought. *Why does this have to be so hard? Haven't I suffered enough?*

I was ushered back over to the hospital and down the same hallways I had walked before. This time, instead of going to the maternity floor, I was told we were headed to the oncology unit.

As the elevator doors opened, faces at the nurses station stopped to stare. I felt like I was on display. The nurse tried telling me that everyone on the floor was great at his or her job and that later someone would show me around and introduce me to the woman who helps people make transitions like wig-fittings and such.

I wanted no part of this new-patient ritual and walked slowly behind thinking, *I don't belong here.* **I DO NOT BELONG HERE!** *This is not happening. I'll show you—I do not belong here! It's all a mistake.*

I was so angry those first couple of hours I don't even remember seeing how Steve and my mom were coping with the news.

I remember a nurse coming in, introducing herself, and promising to take the steps very slowly so I wouldn't be so overwhelmed.

Are you kidding me? I thought.

"That's the most ridiculous thing I've heard yet," I quipped after she left the room. "Let's just get this over with."

A little while later, I heard my mom telling my dad, on the phone, "Well, she's as mad as a hornet."

OK, that's it. "Stop talking about me like I'm not here," I blurted out, as the famous character line from *Steel Magnolias* came to life for me. "Leave me alone. If you're going to call everyone, just do it outside the room. I don't want to talk to anyone and I don't want to hear it over and over," I snapped at her and Steve.

Fury raged inside me because all I wanted to do was just break down and cry. But no tears would come—not that day. Inside I was a wreck. I was afraid of what was about to happen, how long it would go on, and what it all meant for the rest of my life. Was I going to die? Where was the sense in all of this? I couldn't concentrate at all, and I just wanted someone to wake me up when this nightmare was over. I felt as if my life had just entered a drought that was sure to suck out any ounce of life I had left buried below the surface.

I think I pushed enough of my mother's buttons because she and I shared a few cross words with one another. I felt guilty for being so angry; in hindsight, I know I was entitled to my feelings and that they, along with many other emotions, were part of the journey. But I also knew deep down that I was not entitled to treat my family that way. Something inside me snapped and I suddenly realized they were suffering too and were just as helpless as I was. Somehow, I was going to have to pull it together. But I didn't know how.

I was unable to pray. I couldn't even feel Him. I didn't want to talk to Him, even though just the day before I had found myself soaking in the Spirit and felt His peace and protection for my life.

Where are you, God? I quietly wondered.

Later that evening, after a slow series of "steps" and help in getting used to the process, I began the first of what would become weekly chemotherapy treatments. It finally sank in when the nurse entered the room dressed in a full-length rubber gown-like apron, rubber gloves up to her armpits, and a face mask.

Well, isn't this lovely, I thought. *She gets to protect herself from head to toe and I get a mega line directly into my hand and body for this poison."*

Throughout the night, I discovered, she truly was a precious person because she took my searing looks and complete ignoring her all in stride. No matter how mad I was, she remained gracious, kind, and professional (which made me madder, because I felt so stupid for being so selfish).

Dr. Moore, bless his heart, was ever the optimist with my case. But in the early stages, he informed me that he knew for sure the chemotherapy would cause me to lose my hair and make me very sick. He assured me I'd have prescriptions for nausea and mouth sores but to just be prepared.

Hmmmm. I deeply pondered these two side effects. I wasn't crazy about the idea of losing my hair, but I somehow I viewed it as a small sacrifice for my life. In the depths of my soul, I knew I wanted to live and I would endure whatever it took. What frightened me the most, though, was the idea of getting sick.

"Exactly *how* sick will I get?" I asked.

Because I had been so violently ill during the pregnancy, it suddenly became the standard by which I measured "getting sick." Dr. Moore told me everyone responds differently, so there was no way to say in comparison to that yardstick how it would measure up.

I settled in and tried to get used to the idea of these inevitable changes and side effects. By the time the first drop entered my body, I was in survival mode and decided I needed to find some level of acceptance now.

All I knew to hold onto was that Plan A was for sixteen weeks of treatment. So that's what I went with. One step, one week, one treatment at a time.

CHAPTER 18

Interestingly, during the first treatment, I did not get sick while I was in the hospital. I went home with loads of prescriptions, which Steve immediately filled to have ready when the nausea came. Hour by hour we waited for waves of nausea. Nothing.

That first week, Dr. Moore called each day to check on me, and each day I guardedly reported I had not gotten sick. He was pleasantly surprised, but cautiously advised me to still be prepared for it.

For three and a half months, I endured those weekly treatments. One week I'd have to stay overnight in the hospital because that leg of the chemo treatment took about twelve hours to go through the IV. Then the next week, I would go to Dr. Moore's office for a couple of hours for another component of my "cocktail." EMACO was the ordered therapy, and I learned more than I ever dared to imagine possible about each drug component of the therapy.

Days turned into weeks and amazingly, I never got sick. I adored the fact that I finally beat the odds stacked against me in terms of sickness. Not one ounce, not one moment of nausea came upon me. I waited for it, but it never came. We joked about it often but, in my heart, I began to realize that I was being showered by God's mercy. I thanked Him every moment for sparing me from one of my greatest fears at that moment in my life.

The dread of something so horrible had suddenly turned into a promise that I claimed over and over: "But he said to me, 'My grace is sufficient for you, for my power is made perfect in weakness.'..." (2 Corinthians 12:9).

It was late fall, and what our property lacks in terms of a lush green lawn, it certainly makes up for with tall beautiful oaks, maple, pecan, and pine trees. The leaves that had fallen were everywhere. Steve and I were on the road to Jackson for treatments so much that there was little time to do anything about them that year.

As the leaves fell and autumn deepened, I pondered many things about my life, and wondered things that naturally come when someone is faced with the possibility of death. And I discovered a deeper meaning to the fact our property is covered in trees—in particular oaks. I once read in a book, *Streams in the Desert*, that the harder a storm blows, the more the roots of trees deepen. How poignant this metaphor was that was right in my backyard. I found myself watching Steve when he didn't see me and wondered if he'd find joy again. I wondered how my family would cope if I should die. I wondered what legacy would be mine in my community, and I deeply wanted my life to make a difference for someone else's. Admittedly, I was scared I was going to die. I wasn't scared to die, but facing cancer, or any other life-threatening illness, will bring those thoughts to life. For me, they were very real thoughts, but I kept them buried inside. It is not my style to draw attention to myself, and I certainly did not want pity from others while I battled for my life. It's just who I am.

Introspectively, I shared with Steve that I felt like I had entered the "winter" of my life, ironically coinciding with the natural seasons. The images of starkness, dormancy, and retreat were all over the place. And I knew Steve was dealing with the same type of thoughts. But to stay optimistic about my diagnosis and prognosis, we focused on the present. He wouldn't let me get mired down by "what ifs." His defense mechanism was to resist and banish thoughts of dying. In doing so, I learned to live each day for what it brought.

One day, Steve decided we would make the best of our situation, digging beyond the sadness, and take our Christmas card pictures (with Sadie and Lily, of course) smack dab in the middle of the leaves.

I was so excited. Steve knew how much preparing for Christmas meant to me, and taking time to usher the season in was what my soul needed. We showered and dressed in jeans. I chose a red sweater we had gotten the year before in New Zealand. With the self-timer on the camera, we set up the shots in the front yard and managed to get a great family photo that year. I remember being surrounded by my white angels sitting there waiting for Steve to mash the timer button and thinking, *This may be the last Christmas picture we ever take.* I didn't want everything I did or said to be so gloom and doom, but I couldn't help but be a little nostalgic.

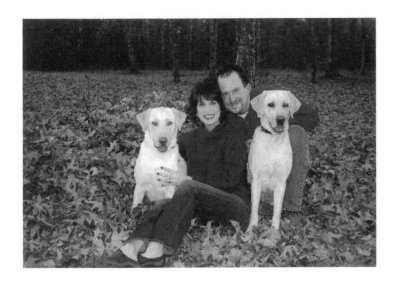

Our 2003 Christmas photo.

I don't know what came over me that day, but in the instant the camera started flashing, my heart lit up as well. Time became more about making the most of the moments I had left—whether they were limited to a few months or fifty more years. The place where I had always gone deep inside myself for strength had been slowly dwindling, but I suddenly found myself reaching even further and coming up with a daily handful and heart full of renewal. I explained it to my mother as floating along on a cloud of grace.

To try and explain this epiphany is quite difficult. Some don't understand it at all—they want explanations of how I got to this place of peace. I see it more as a series of seasons throughout my life that had finally cultivated in that moment. To miss this lesson is to miss the entire purpose of this book. We are brought into and through times in our lives purposefully.

It may take months, years even, to understand the whys and hows. In fact, those answers may never come at all. But it's the fruits of what has been planted that we focus on. What we do with intended lessons is in direct relationship to where we end up in our lives.

Over and over, day by day, promises flooded my soul and began to water the cracks and crevices of my life. I spent a lot of time writing notes and cards to friends and family. I wrote more in my journal during those months than I had ever written in my life. I spent a lot of time praying and reading scripture and began the intimate journey of getting to know Christ. I had been saved early in my life, but I finally got what if felt like to work on a personal relationship with Him.

Peace. Sweet peace. And there it was for the taking. On many days, I did not know how things would turn out at the end of the road, but I knew God promised me peace. That's all I had. At the end of each day, peace was in my heart.

Peace I leave with you; my peace I give you. I do not give to you as the world gives. Do not let your hearts be troubled and do not be afraid.

John 14:27

CHAPTER 19

I have to admit that while I knew my hair would grow back after treatments, I was a little nervous about the possibility of losing it. Anyone who has been through chemotherapy encounters the "what ifs" along the way. *What if I wake up and my hair stays on my pillow? What if it grows back differently? What if I look ugly?* To help soften the blow, Steve had already been planning a "shave the head" day for himself when the time came. We laughed and joked about being the two bald Browns around town, but I could not see myself with no hair. I just couldn't visualize it—not because I was in denial about it happening, but because I mentally could not get a picture.

In retrospect, it seems quite vain to even give a moment's dignity to those questions or concerns. But we are human, and I was certainly more than a little concerned. I did not talk about it much, because I did not want everyone to think of me as vain. There's not a vain bone in my body, but as women, our hair helps define our personalities, our femininity, and our identity as we see ourselves in the mirrors.

I know that other women feel an attachment to their hair as well. One day I went to my salon for a nail appointment with my manicurist, Pam. She and my hairdresser brought over a gift bag. As I opened it, my heart sank in complete humility.

There in the bottom of the bag was a beautiful mass of brown hair. Together they had purchased a beautiful wig for me—ready to be styled just like my hair. It was there, ready for me for the day when I would need it. It was just the nurturing I needed, an added bit of nourishment and encouragement to keep facing the sun and walking through the valley. I knew I was not alone in my thoughts about my hair and the Lord used that moment in time for those precious women and friends to minister to me in a way that was unspeakable for me to that point.

I arrived home that same afternoon to find a package left on my front door step. I opened the beautifully wrapped box and inside was the cutest black crushed velvet hat that had been dropped off with a note from a high school friend of Steve's.

Weeks went by with more chemotherapy treatments, and although it began to thin some, the majority of my hair remained in my head. It was such a marvel that even the hospital pharmacist came down to visit me during one of my stays to make sure what he was hearing about me was true. I still had my hair!

I received two more shipped packages from my sister— beautiful hats she had ordered for me. Additionally, my chamber of commerce colleagues from across the Southeast began a hat campaign. Each person from my U.S. Chamber of Commerce Institute class sent me a hat representing his or her community. In all, I have a great collection of ball caps, an Arkansas Razorback foam head, and a sun cap from the Tour de France!

Once again, God knew my heart and my fears, and without my having to cry over it or talk about it with our friends and family, he used others to support and encourage me in just the way I needed—just when I needed it. And one of my fears and worries was no longer a concern.

Indeed, the very hairs of your head are all numbered.
Don't be afraid; you are worth more than many sparrows.

Luke 12:7

CHAPTER 20

Exhaustion is one of the side effects of chemotherapy, and I was exhausted a lot. I continued working except on the days of my treatments. Most days I worked until 1 or 2 p.m. or until I would hit the proverbial "brick wall" and could no longer stand up. I would work as long as I could each day and then I would go home and sleep every afternoon until Steve got home from work. Some days we had meals that people had generously provided for us. Other days we cooked together. When friends offered to bring us food, I had to learn to accept their offers graciously. We had offers for household help from many friends and family, but I am such the independent person, I wanted to maintain as much normalcy in my life as possible. That is important to many cancer patients.

The independent side of me that developed so early in my life wanted no part of pity from anyone. I wanted others to treat me as they always had. Just because I was now living with cancer, it didn't change *who* I was. I experienced what it meant to be lifted up in prayer. I could honestly feel prayers over my life in a way I had never known before. And the ability to get through each day made me realize it was nothing that I was doing—it was much more than being about me. It was grace.

I learned the importance of taking care of my health and listening to what my body needed. I knew better than to shake hands with business associates and I had to avoid crowds because my immune system was compromised by the chemotherapy.

Each week before I could have my chemotherapy, we had to know where my white and red cell counts were. If the counts are too low, the treatment has to be delayed until they are at an acceptable level. So we would drive to our family physician's office on the way to Jackson for a CBC check. Early on, the coast was clear. But eventually, the chemo took its toll and we hit a place that my white cell counts were too low.

I had to go further to Jackson anyway to begin an every-other-week series of shots of Neulasta and Procrit to boost white blood cell and red blood cell counts, respectively. Once I started these treatments, I became even more aware of how tired I had become. I actually looked forward to receiving the shots to boost my red and white cell counts because I knew I needed energy and stamina, and I needed to continue with my treatments.

To keep my spirits up, a small group of my chamber of commerce colleagues planned a road trip to Starkville, Mississippi, to visit me. They came from North Carolina, Texas, Georgia, and parts of Mississippi to visit me one weekend. I introduced them to our small university town, and we laughed so hard the entire weekend. Having people drive for hours and hours just to see you as you go through a difficult time is something everyone should experience. I was, at that time, totally amazed—not surprised—but amazed that these very busy people, who have families and careers of their own, would take time to come and cheer up a friend. They drove for hours to get to me. These special people will forever have a special place in my heart and their never-ending calls, cards, hats, and notes of encouragement taught me how to be a better friend and colleague.

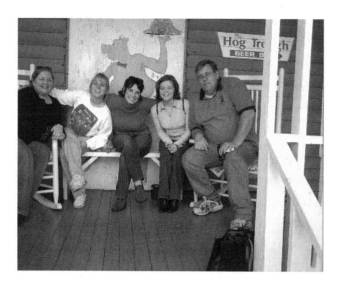

Chamber friends, Beth, Abbie, Kristi, Hilary, Allen

My progress was measured each week by my HCG levels. Slowly each week they descended until they finally plateaued. It appeared the chemotherapy was no longer working and Plan B became apparent. By mid-January, I was scheduled for a PET scan—a high-powered, slow-moving scan over every part of the body. I was injected intravenously with radioactive fluid and was ordered to lie still on a gurney for an hour to allow the fluid to permeate throughout my body. I thought it was going to be hard to relax thinking about a radioactive serum being pumped inside me, but I managed to pass the time dreaming of a massage and imagining I was on the beach with the waves crashing on the shore just below my feet.

After the scan results came back, we realized we needed a change of course. The lesions on my lung and liver were no longer showing up. What a blessing! But the news was bittersweet, because the scan showed one tumor that remained in my uterus.

I'll never forget the day I realized surgery was inevitable. I was alone in my hospital room, as Steve had driven to Meridian to make some sales calls for work. Dr. Moore entered and, as he was leaning against the window, he began retracing the steps we had taken over the past few months. He had waited as long as he could to preserve the opportunity for us to try to get pregnant again.

I broke the silence and spoke up. "Dr. Moore, if you're waiting on me to give you permission to do a hysterectomy, it's time. Steve and I have discussed it, and if that's what we have to do, we are ready."

I couldn't believe I was hearing those words come from my mouth. They hovered around the hospital room for what seemed like an eternity. But Dr. Moore looked relieved. I had saved him from having to tell me himself that we were facing Plan B. Plan A was no longer working. I was tired, yet I was ready.

In my heart I knew the door for us to have a baby was not only closed, it was now necessary that it be locked.

Hysterectomy. That was Plan B.

I Still Believe (by Jeremy Camp)*

Scattered words and empty thoughts
Seem to pour from my heart
I've never felt so torn before
Seems I don't know where to start
But it's now that I feel your grace fall like rain
From every fingertip washing away my pain

I still believe in your faithfulness
I still believe in your truth
I still believe in your holy word
Even when I don't see, I still believe

Though the questions still fog up my mind
With promises I still seem to bear
Even when answers slowly unwind
It's my heart I see you prepare
But its now, that I feel, your grace fall like rain
From every fingertip washing away my pain

I still believe in your faithfulness
I still believe in your truth
I still believe in your holy word
Even when I don't see, I still believe

Well the only place I can go is into your arms
Where I throw to you my feeble prayers well in brokenness
I can see that this was your will for me
Help me to know that you are near

I still believe in your faithfulness
I still believe in your truth
I still believe in your holy word
Even when I don't see, I still believe

I still believe
Ohhh, I still believe, I still believe

CHAPTER 21

I had only a couple of days to get prepared for surgery. I took leave from work, sent e-mails to friends and family, boarded Sadie and Lily, and packed my bags.

Once more I checked into the hospital and went through the series of questions, blood work, and prep time. Finally, I was wheeled into the operating room for what we hoped would put an end to what I had been diagnosed with as gestational trophoblast disease (GTD). Surgery was predictable and went well. But even after removing both ovaries and my uterus, my HCG levels continued to stay positive. It puzzled us all, Dr. Moore included. And I found myself a week after surgery traveling back to Jackson for more chemotherapy. Plan C. Sometimes life moves more swiftly than we wish and my choices were zooming by. I was tired—emotionally and physically. My body was not the same and had not been for a long time. I could not believe that after every bit of my female organs had been surgically removed, my body was still indicating a high HCG.

After two additional weeks of chemo, Dr. Moore decided we would take a "wait and see" approach to following my HCG levels to a negative number. Though they were not considered to be negative, they were low enough to be able to back off of chemo. I continued to travel to Jackson every couple of weeks to check my HCGs.

And finally, in April of 2004 I was given an "all clear" from a CT scan. "Cancer free" never sounded so good to me.

Within a couple of months, I celebrated with a trip to a spa, and Steve threw me a "Survivor"-themed party complete with a band, family and friends, and Dr. Moore.

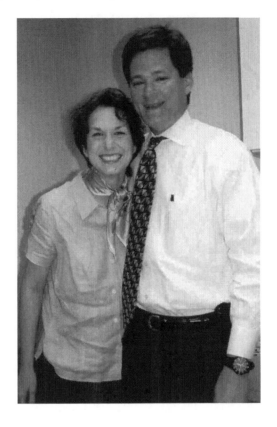

Dr. Moore and me the day I received my first "all clear" scan.

"If you, even you, had only known on this day what would bring you peace—but now it is hidden from your eyes."

Luke 19:42

CHAPTER 22

So how does one finally come to peace with closed doors? Although we always dreamed we would have a family, Steve and I have come to realize that having children is not the pinnacle of who we are as a couple or as individuals. It is not the summit of our lives. More importantly, it is not the plan for our lives.

Additionally, I firmly believe that going through all that I went through did not define me; it refined me. Once diagnosed with GTD, I joined an elite group of individuals who face and fight cancer every single day of their lives. Locally, my community has an incredibly close-knit group of individuals who "just know" what it means not only to live with it but also to live through it. One of my favorite quotes by Italian dramatist and poet Vittorio Alfieri best sums it up: "Often the test of courage is not to die but to live." And while I do not want to walk down that path again, I wouldn't take a million dollars for what I have learned and who I have become.

My life was broken apart, dug into, tilled up, fertilized, pollinated, watered, broken again, pollinated, and watered again so much that I understand that we all have these seasons in our lives that create what we call our lives. It is our choice day by day what we do with these gardens. It is our responsibility to take care of ourselves emotionally, physically, and spiritually so that we may become more than a dormant spot of weeds.

I have learned that our trials are purposeful and

intentional. Our blessings are very evident in the lives we choose to live, although our culture does not readily recognize or understand couples who have no children, either by choice or by circumstance. In fact, some people border on being absolutely rude and nosey; we all can learn to be more selective and less intrusive about asking personal questions.

Through my experiences, I have learned to help those who have been blessed with the precious gifts of children to be sensitive to those who haven't. I will not purposefully embark upon others' personal lives by asking couples if they have children.

Though it has taken several years, I've learned to smile when Steve and I are asked if we have children. I've learned that we all take things for granted—even pregnant moms-to-be who flippantly complain about gaining weight or being tired. I've learned that I can send gifts for baby showers rather than feeling like I must show up in person. I've come to accept that others are still learning that they don't have to "fix" Steve and me by suggesting we adopt or asking us if we are ever going to adopt.

The lesson in this is that we are not all meant to live in the same way. Our gifts to the world are decided by a much Higher Power than how we perceive they should be used.

Just like every spot on this journey I've found myself on, God has again revealed himself to me. And as I am finishing this book—just today driving home, in this glorious springtime season—His Promises are once again laid out in front of me like the way the sunlight dances just in front of my car. I can never quite catch it, but it is always there—one step in front of, beside, or behind me.

Sometimes the lessons of life are taught to us in ways that make us long to be rescued. The droughts are often long;

parts of the garden are often stunted in growth and filled with weeds; the flowers die and need to be de-headed and cut back. We often need different fertilizers, more or less water, wind, and sun. But the harvest is plenty.

The revelation for our hardships, our trials, our joys, our hurts, and victories in these times is our calling and we all have purposeful seasons in life. Yes, I may be physically infertile, but my life is not. I may not have children of my own to carry on an earthly family heritage, or to be an extension of my family tree, but my riches, my harvest, and my eternal family have been stored up in Heaven.

In the same way, your trials are but for a moment. They are intended to ground you, to prune you, and to make you a beautiful living example for others.

CHAPTER 23

Like all cancer survivors, my journey never really ends. Even a few years later, I am followed closely with regular visits to check my levels. I was recently reminded that it hasn't been that long ago since we finally saw my HCG levels drop to a negative number.

Looking back, even at my darkest hour, I felt the Holy Spirit fill my soul and body, as I had never experienced it before. God truly gave me the grace to endure what He had in store for me.

I've learned that what some would call a tragedy, I call a "divine time out" (thank you, Mom). I cannot begin to tell you how or when I knew the Lord was in the midst of all of this, but my faith has taught me that we are not meant to have all the answers and that our plans for our own lives are not always what He plans.

I am too weak and imperfect to fix me. I finally learned to accept the fact that the Lord not only shut the door on our having a baby, but he locked it forever. Closed doors in our lives sometimes hurt. But I know that in the midst of all things good and bad, God is still on His throne. Our greatest hurts can become our greatest blessings.

I am grateful to be surrounded with family, friends, a caring community, and people all over this country that I do not even know who have prayed for us through the long roads of heartache. I have never experienced anything like the presence of the Holy Spirit as I did during those dark, dark moments of my life. But just as the earth needs both night and day, we need those same moments to grow us into an awakened garden.

As that self-proclaimed transitional person I realized I was earlier in my life, I made it my mission to face every day with all the zest of life that God could allow someone to have. And I now know that every step of my life, whether in heartbreak or in joy, has been in preparation for moments that I know will produce a harvest from which others glean.

Because of the journey I've been on—including and especially the darkest moments—I have been able to discover my passion and live out and up to the dreams I have had for a very long time. The personal growth and reflections on my life have given me the courage and faith to step out and start a new business, write a book, encourage others, and bloom—living life to the fullest.

Choosing to live a fertile life does not come in a petri dish. It's not measured in the number of children one has, the accomplishments listed on a resume, or the amount of money one acquires.

A fertile life grows in the soul. It's born of integrity, courage, faith, and dreams. Fertile living is the pouring out of yourself so that others may grow. It is learning to accept that which we do not understand and rising above that which seeks to stunt our growth. A fertile life blooms proliferately after seasons of tilling, planting, fertilizing, pruning, and nourishment.

The lessons are simple really. Plant wisely. Take care of your life's garden. There are blessings to claim from any heartbreak or heartache. An abundant life springs forth from a well-watered, fertilized, tilled, pruned, and wisely seeded life.

To choose joy over despair, right over wrong, humility over pride, and to have faith in the unseen—these are the steps one must begin to take to walk on fertile ground.

He will be like a tree planted by the water
that sends out its roots by the stream.
It does not fear when heat comes;
its leaves are always green.
It has no worries in a year of drought and
never fails to bear fruit.

Jeremiah 17:8